PREFACE

Thank you for purchasing "BUD BASICS" the first book in the INFO IS POWER series produced by Green Irene @ Cannabis Corner Café. This publication is **not** a definitive, all inclusive resource by any stretch of the imagination.   It is, however, a compendium of basic general knowledge gathered and presented by its author, Irene A York who continues to pour over research studies old and new, chipping away at the archaic attitudes and associative stigmas associated with cannabis and its consumption or use.

NOTE FROM THE AUTHOR

With the belief that **normalization** of cannabis will free the leaf far more powerfully and effectively than any legalization or legislation can, I continue to study the "Sciences" behind cannabis and its consumption.

After decades of prohibition and demonization of this wonderful weed, it's true nature can **finally be revealed!** Education is empowering, and acceptance of the herb has come at long last *(for the most part)*. Pot is no longer a dirty little secret, to be consumed furtively and hidden from friends, family or co-workers. Cannabis is going mainstream and for millions of North Americans – this is GREAT news.

Seasoned consumers and newbies alike can enjoy and reap the benefits that Cannabis can provide without fear of discrimination, ostracization or persecution. However, as this writer has learned – there is a lot of MIS information as well as missing information on the subject, and through this series - **INFO IS POWER**, I intend to share the mountains of research I've gathered. Subscribe to www.cannabiscornercafe.ca / www.greenirene.ca to receive up to date information on guest appearances, live presentations, workshops and more. GREEN IRENE is on the scene; providing answers or guidance to the climbing number of CANNABIS CURIOSITIES – EMPOWERING MY AUDIENCES WITH INFORMATION – ARMING INDIVIDUALS WITH TOOLS FOR SUCCESSFUL STRATEGY IMPLEMENTATION – GIVING EVERY PATIENT THE AUTHORITY TO TAKE RESPONSIBILITY FOR THE QUALITY OF THEIR HEALTH, WELLNESS & HAPPINESS.

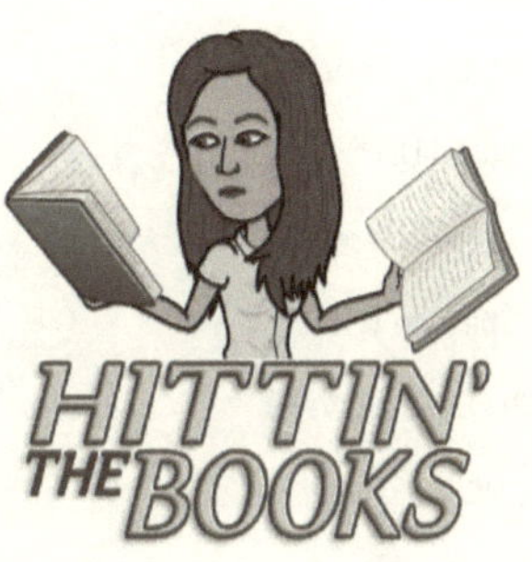

Contents

BUD BASICS

INTRODUCTION

Cannabis is a popular topic these days thanks to the cascade of cannabis law reform around the globe. Since most confusion surrounding the plant, is the result of misinformation, missing information and lies spread by prohibitionists for the past eight to ten decades – the subject can be quite daunting, and curiosities remain uncured ….

This book is designed to help answer some of the common curiosities providing a rudimentary basic understanding for the Cannabis Newbie. Directions and links to additional information and resources are made available at points of interest and should be followed if you'd like a deeper understanding of a specific topic.

Beginning with the most basic curiosity *"What is the difference between cannabis, pot, marijuana (sometimes spelt – marihuana) weed, ganga, bhang, dope etc.?"*

In short, all the terms reference the CANNABIS Plant from which thousands upon thousands of strains, with very different and unique traits can be identified based on the family of genetics it's derived from – *namely,* SATIVA – INDICA -RUDERALIS

Although sativa, Indica and ruderalis are 3 very distinct and different families of cannabis, they are interbreedable. Which essentially means that there are many strains that possess the qualities of multiple families and are commonly called Hybrids. The benefit of hybridization is that the breeder can attempt to create strains that are profiled to specific wants and needs.

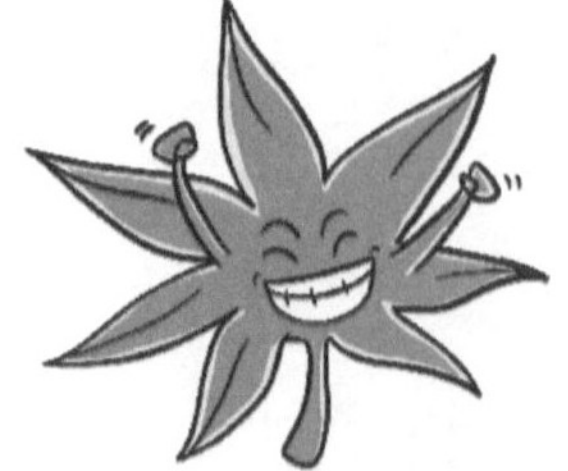

In today's market hybrid strains dominate the market, as most strains have been crossed at one time or another. Understanding the difference between these genetic families can help growers and consumers make informed decisions.

CANNABIS SATIVA

Sativa strains are physically the largest. They originated in the wilds of equatorial countries primarily between 30 degrees North and 30 degrees south of the equator. In these equatorial countries, the hours of daylight do not fluctuate throughout the year in the same way it does across the rest of the globe. Cannabis sativa plants have evolved to take advantage of this and continue to grow as they flower reaching heights of up to 20 feet in a single season. The leaves of the cannabis sativa plant are long and spindly, often described as being finger-like – much like the stereotypical representation of a cannabis leaf. Flavors range from earthy to sweet and fruity.

Pure sativa cannabis is a challenge to cultivate in the northern hemisphere (Canada) and seeds are hard to come by. Although pure Sativas are quite rare, they are highly coveted by breeders who use their genetic stability to create designer hybrid strains. Cannabis sativa plants tend to have very high concentrations of THC and relatively low levels of CBD, which has been further strengthened by human breeding.

When you consume a sativa strain you might feel energized, thoughtful, focused, generally awesome and uplifted, with a stimulated head high. Sativas also have a lighter, fruitier aroma. In other words, if you want to be social, clean your house, have brilliant ideas, or manage to accomplish anything at all, Sativas are your go-to. Sativas are also wonderful for physical activities and Rocky Mountain adventures. Inhalation or ingestion of pure sativa typically produces an "uplifting high" that can be characterized in the following ways...

- Cerebral "heady" buzz
- Energizing / uplifted mood
- Motivation
- Focus/increased alertness
- Inspiration / increased creativity
- Helps relieve depression / promotes a sense of wellbeing
- Stimulates the appetite and helps to reduce nausea

However, the negative effects of too much pure sativa can induce paranoia and irregular heart beats much like too much caffeine, making "PURE SATIVA" a rare choice when used strictly for medicinal reasons. Unlike Sativa Hybrids!

Sativa Hybrid

A hybrid sativa dominant strain is coveted as medicine for the motivational properties they possess. They tend to be uplifting and produce an energetic cerebral high without the paranoia. The sativa strains are cross pollinated to fit special criteria such as smell, taste and stimulant effect.

CANNABIS INDICA

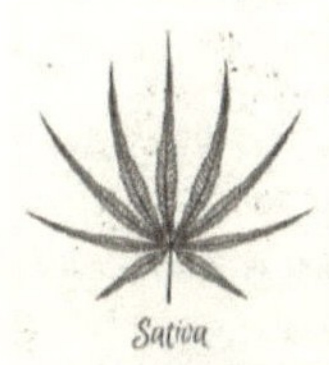

Pure Indica's originally come from the sub-tropical hash producing countries of the world like Pakistan, Afghanistan, Morocco and Tibet. They are short, dense plants, with broad fan like leaves that often grow a darker green, with more chlorophyll and less accessory pigments (accessory pigments protect the plant from excessive sunlight) the fingers of the leaves tend to grow much wider. Once the plants reach their ideal height, they put all their energy into producing flowers. After flowering starts, they will mature in 6 to 8 weeks (much sooner than Sativas) and are better for indoor growing because they do not grow as tall as Sativas. The flowers will be thick and dense, with flavors and aromas ranging from pungent skunk to sweet and fruity.

Indica plants have by far the most pain fighting, sedating and relaxing effect. Cannabis Indica strains are known for having a much higher CBD content than Sativas. One of the many functions of CBD is to moderate the effect THC has on the body and mind. Thus, Indica strains have a very different effect than Sativas. These effects include:

- A body buzz
- Acting as a muscle relaxant
- Reduces inflammation

- Effective pain relief/management
- Aids sleep
- Acting as a sedative
- Increasing the appetite
- Increasing dopamine production
- Relieving stress and anxiety

Patients usually use indicas for insomnia and severe pain later in the day as it has a strong cloudy type of high. Their strong sedating and pain blocking qualities are highly coveted by medical patients.

Hybrid Indica Dominant

In terms of medical value these are the best and most widely appreciated. Today's "Kush" strains are a prime example of these types and are easily the most popular among recreational and medical consumers. These strains tend to have many qualities that both grower and consumer find to their liking, therefore most of medical cannabis is hybrid Indica. Notably, they are helpful as a sleeping aid for those suffering from injury, insomnia or severe inflammation.

CANNABIS HYBRID

Hybrids can be broken down into three basic categories:

1. Sativa-dominant Hybrids: Cerebral high with a relaxing body effect. Can provide both mental and physical relief. Strains include: Glass Slipper, Super Lemon Haze, Lemon Skunk

2. Even Hybrids (50/50): Ideal strains for people seeking a balanced euphoria of head and body relaxation. Strains include: Pineapple Express, Super Silver Haze, Blueberry Headband

3. Indica-dominant Hybrids: These strains may provide full-body pain relief and mitigation, with a relaxing head euphoria. Usually used in the afternoon and nighttime, beneficial for sleep. These strains may be ideal for patients who suffer from all types of autoimmune diseases as well as insomnia and depression. Strains include: Kosher Tangie, Dark Blue Dream, Brownie Scout

CANNABIS RUDERALIS

This is a relatively new line/family of the cannabis plant typically found growing wild in colder regions (like Russia & China) The main feature of the ruderalis family is that it is *autoflowering* - which means it flowers based on age not light schedule – translation, the cultivator has less conditions to be concerned about or responsible for. Ruderalis has very little THC content and is hardly, if ever grown for recreational purposes. Its high content of CBD (Cannabidiol) is making it increasingly popular as breeding stock for medicinal strains.

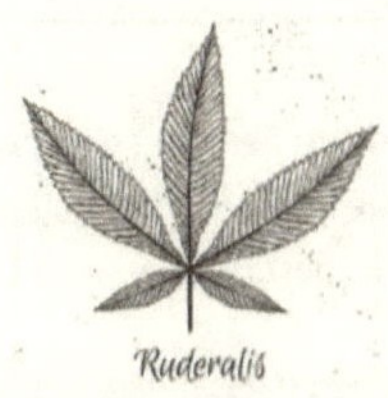

Ruderalis

When cross bred with an indica or sativa the plant will very likely produce a strain that is both autoflowering and higher in CBD content. Ruderalis strains are also very small and very fast growing. They produce very small leaves and only a few side branches. Additionally, it is quite resistant to damage by insects or disease. This is a huge advantage for many growers, especially those who live in colder areas of the world, and/or those who grow outdoors. For all intent purposes, it means a crop can be planted, maintained with little effort and then replanted right after harvest – as flowering will be affected by time growing as opposed to seasonal change.

Cannabis ruderalis and its genetic/medical benefits has drastically changed the way geneticists and seed breeders are creating strains which is rapidly changing the industry. Overall, ruderalis has very low levels of THC & CBD, rendering them worthless to use in pure form; however, when bred with sativa or indica strains it is possible to produce an indica/sativa dominant plant with autoflowering genetics.

Summarily, although sativa, indica and ruderalis are three very distinct and different families of cannabis, hybridization from cross breeding has produced some really stunning results. Check out leafly.com – the self-proclaimed largest database of strain information.

*Since the first publication of BUD BASICS – several other **STRAIN DATABASE** websites have emerged – **SEE UPDATED REFERENCES***

HEMP *or* CANNABIS Sativa L

Hemp is one of the oldest domesticated crops known to man. It has been used for paper, textiles, and cordage for thousands of years, in fact the oldest relic of human industry is a scrap of hemp fabric dating back to approximately 8,000 BC. Its the single greatest plant resource for human health and well being – food, clothing, shelter, medicine. Hemp plants are naturally found on all continents. There are many different varieties of the cannabis plant. Hemp — also called industrial hemp — referring to the non-psychoactive (less than 1% THC) varieties of Cannabis Sativa L. Both hemp and marijuana *(a slang term) come* from the

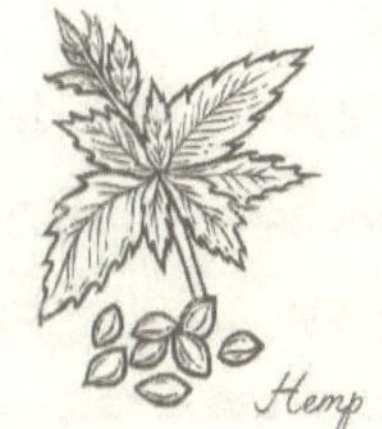

Hemp

same cannabis species but are genetically distinct and are further distinguished by use, chemical makeup, and cultivation methods.

Hemp can be grown as a renewable source for raw materials that can be incorporated into thousands of products. Its seeds and flowers are used in health foods, organic body care, and other nutraceuticals. It is one of the most essential nutrient dense and balanced foods available and provides an excellent easily digestible source of protein and balanced good fats for human health.

Hemp is an attractive rotation crop for farmers. As it grows, hemp breathes in CO2, detoxifies the soil, and prevents soil erosion. What's left after harvest breaks down into the soil, providing valuable nutrients. It requires much less water to grow — and little if any chemical fertilizers, fungicides, herbicides or pesticides — so it is much more environmentally friendly than traditional crops.

Many factors have helped contribute to the recent rapid increase in hemp use and production. More and more consumers have come to appreciate the nutritional and health benefits of hemp. Manufacturers are recognizing the many uses—new and old—of hemp fibres. They see the value of a strong, versatile fibre that is relatively inexpensive, completely renewable and environmentally beneficial.

Hemp can do a lot, but it can't get you "high." Because hemp varieties contain virtually zero tetrahydrocannabinol (THC), your body processes it faster than you can smoke it, besides which, the burnt plant material and associative carcinogens will likely produce or result in a rather unpleasant headache.

Ask anyone passionate about the benefits of hemp, and they will tell you about the hemp car produced by Henry Ford in 1941. According to the lore, it was made entirely out of hemp-based plastics and had an engine built to run on hemp fuel. The New York Post, from the Henry Ford Museum itself, and a youtube video are now easily accessible to those seeking more information.

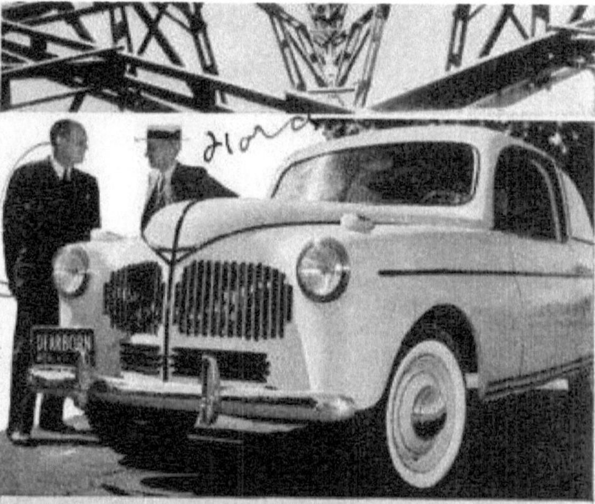

Here is the auto Henry Ford "grew from the soil." Its plastic panels, with impact strength 10 times greater than steel, were made from flax, wheat, hemp, spruce pulp

urers are seeking substitutes nearly like the originals as pos- e. Neckties of spun glass are beautiful as those of silk, may st wrinkling even better. Plas- tips for shoestrings released ut a half million pounds of als, principally tin, to more ll industries in 1941 alone and never knew the difference. ig before the emergency shut n silk supplies, du Pont chem- magicians had plucked out of air, the sea and the coal mine elements of nylon, and mills ricating nylon hosiery were anding rapidly; and govern- it research men were develop- lovely new designs for cotton

(Continued to page 201)

CANNABIS JARGON

Being new to the cannabis culture is made more daunting and confusing by some of the technical, medical and scientific terms and acronyms commonly used as part of the associative jargon. So, here is a basic overview of the most frequently used terms and a brief explanation of what they mean...

- Cannabinoid: These are the chemical compounds gleaned from the cannabis plant that give the 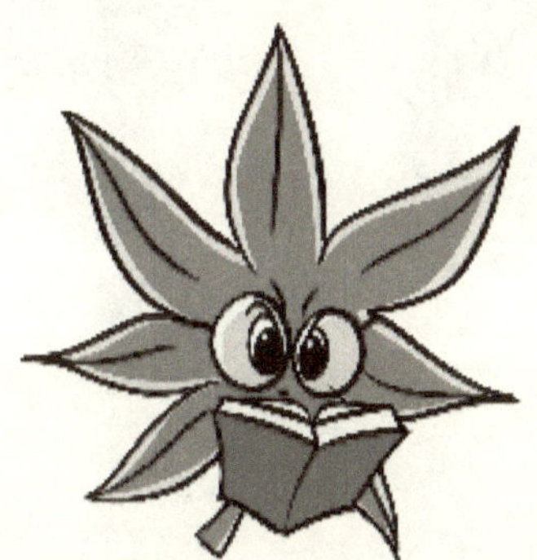 cannabis its medical and recreational properties. The most well known of which are THC and CBD, though there are many researched and studied. See the list of references and resources for a more information.

  o **THC**: *short for tetrahydrocannabinol or delta9-Tetrahydrocannabinol, which is one of the more than 80 cannabinoids in cannabis. It is the principal psychoactive component of cannabis. THC binds to cannabis receptors and kick-starts a series of chemical reactions that causes changes in the brain and in the body. When THC engages your brain, you will experience altered cognitive and behavioral ability. In other words, THC is what causes the cerebral "high" when you consume cannabis through inhalation or ingestion.*

  o **CBD**: *short for cannabidiol. It is another cannabinoid found in cannabis. CBD is non-psychoactive. In fact, it can counter the psychoactive effects of THC. Unlike THC which directly binds to cannabinoid receptors, CBD does not engage the same receptors that well. Instead, CBD inhibits the production of the enzyme FAAHm which breaks down an endocannabinoid called anandamide. Anandamine increases the natural endocannabinoids in our system. CBD, as a result, allows the endocannabinoids to flourish and makes it available for our cells to use. This is the reason why CBD has mood-lifting effects, among many health benefits.*

- **CBC, CBG, CBN** are a couple that I have researched a little more extensively. Information about how and why they apply to a positive health and wellness strategy is related throughout the series INFO IS POWER as the information applies.

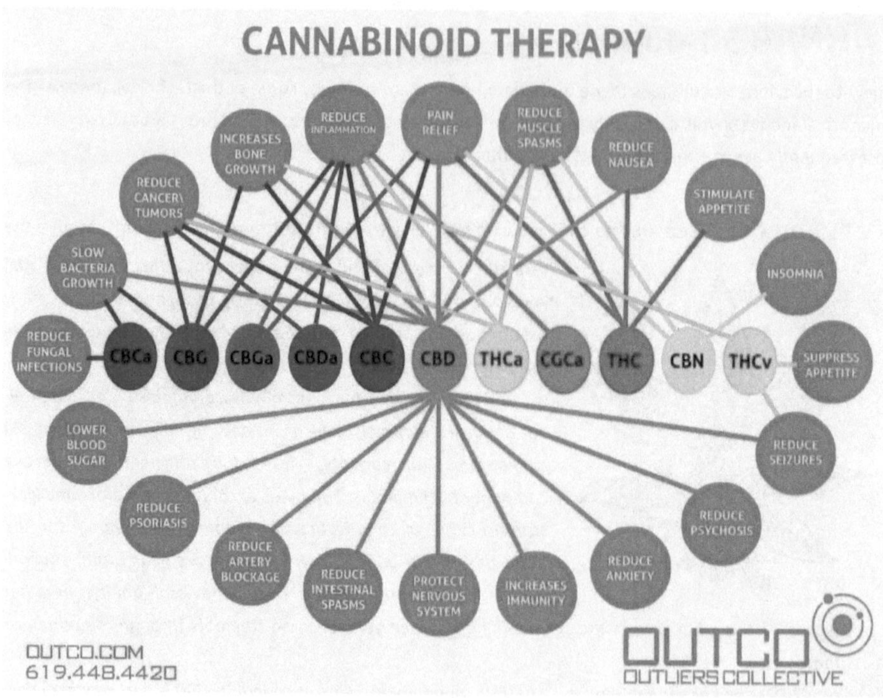

Image Source: http://outcoca.blogspot.ca/2014/12/the-medicinal-properties-of-cannabinoids.html

Cannabinoids interact with the cannabinoid receptors found in our body's cells producing a range of effects.

Simply put, cannabinoids are the chemical messengers for our endocannabinoid system or **ECS** for short.

The human endocannabinoid system is responsible for maintaining our body's balance or state of homeostasis, and regulating many of the body's basic functions, including appetite, pain response, metabolism, sleep, movement, mood, memory and learning, temperature, immune response, inflammation, neuroprotection, neural development, digestion, cardiovascular function, and even reproduction.

It is an amazing biological system that is a collection of endocannabinoids or neurotransmitters that bind to or activate cannabinoid receptors. Metabolic enzymes break down the endocannabinoids after they've been used. **Simply put, the ECS has three key components: cannabinoid receptors, endocannabinoids or neurotransmitters, and metabolic enzymes.**

Cannabinoid Receptors

Cannabis receptors are located on the surface of cells - basically, waiting for messages, listening for a change conditions outside of the cells and transmit that information to the inside of these cells, so that the cells know what to to do! This means that cannabinoids are the messengers and cannabinoid receptors are the message receivers. There are currently 2 types of cannabinoid receptors studied in the human body.

They are known as CB1 and CB2.

- **CB1:** This is one of two major types of cannabinoid receptors. CB1 receptors can be found throughout the body, but they are concentrated in the brain and in the central nervous system. They are mainly found in regions of the brain that are associated with appetite regulation and emotional and memory processing. They are also found in abundance in nerve endings, where they act to lessen the sensations of pain.

- **CB2:** This is the other major type of cannabinoid receptors. CB2 receptors are mainly expressed in our immune system and in our hematopoietic cells (blood cells). The gastrointestinal tract hosts a large amount of CB2 receptors as does the peripheral nervous system. When CB2 receptors are activated, they reduce inflammation.

Titration:

The more scientific name for "try-and-see" practice is **titration**. You'll often hear this term bandied around by those in the know because it's easier to say than, "the process of trial and error by which you determine the right amount of cannabis that your unique endocannabinoid system requires in order to feel optimal." Why say 26 words when you can say just one and mean the same thing? Start using the word titration now!

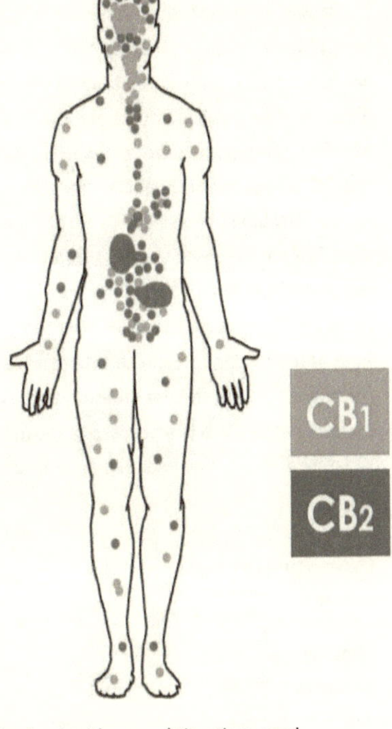

DECARBOXYLATION – *how and why*

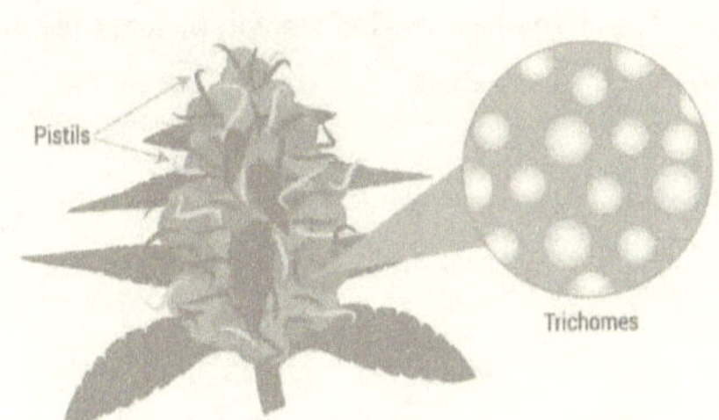

Decarboxylation Explained

It basically means the removal or loss of a carboxyl group from an organic compound. In the case of weed, this would simply mean "losing or removing" the acid compound.

All cannabinoids are produced and stored in the trichomes of the plant – the trichomes are the crystals that "*sugar coat*" the leaves, buds and stalk – it is typically a sticky substance. As these cannabinoids are produced and stored they have an extra carboxyl ring or group (COOH) attached to their chain of molecules. For example, THC (tetrahydrocannabinol) is produced and stored as tetrahydrocannabinolic acid (THCA). THCA has many known health and wellness benefits, including neuroprotective qualities but due to the extra molecule, (COOH), will NOT attach to the cannabinoid receptors in our brain that produce the euphoric effect of *"being high"*.

DECARBOXYLATION is the process of removing the extra molecule. There are two means by which the molecular conversion can happen – heat and time.   Drying or curing the cannabis flowers over time will generate a partial decarboxylation. Adding heat (or heating the product) will instantaneously decarboxylate cannabinoids. Vaporizing/Combustion converts cannabinoids immediately due to the extremely high temperatures present, making them instantly available for absorption through inhalation.

While decarboxylated cannabinoids in vapor form can be easily absorbed in our lungs, edibles require decarboxylated cannabinoids present in what we consume to achieve full absorption.

At What Temperature Does Decarboxylation Occur?

The THCA in cannabis begins to decarboxylate at approximately 200-220 degrees Fahrenheit after around 30-45 minutes of exposure. Full decarboxylation may require more time to occur. Many people choose to decarboxylate their cannabis at slightly lower temperatures for a much longer period in attempts to preserve terpenes. The integrity of both cannabinoids and terpenoids are compromised by using temperatures that exceed 300 degrees F, which is why temperatures in the 200's is recommended.

Heat and time can also cause other forms of cannabinoid degradation to occur. For example, CBN (cannabinol) is formed through the degradation and oxidization of THC – in other words, stale weed that's been hanging around awhile! This is a process that can occur alongside decarboxylation. CBN accounts for a much more sedative and less psychoactive experience.

Decarboxylation Methods:

Tip: Grind or chop up your cannabis first, it allows your weed to evenly dry without losing potency from over grinding.

Flower/Keif/Hash

Preheat your oven according to the chart provided (225F-300F) on average.

Sprinkle your cannabis in a pie plate and then cover it well with silver foil by crimping the foil along the edge of the plate.

Place in the oven – less time for older drier material, more for fresher material.

After required time, turn the oven off, and remove cannabis. Let it cool down slowly before you unseal the container to allow any cannabinoid/terpenes vapor to reabsorb into the cannabis.

Boiling Bag method:

Place the cannabis flower/keif/hash into a boilable cooking pouch. Seal it.

Place in boiling water for 90 minutes. Make sure water does not boil dry.

Take bag out of water. Let it slowly cool before opening.

Cannabis Oil

Place heat proof container of cannabis oil into a cooking oil bath (canola oil works well). Heat cooking oil to 121C/250F.

Stir cannabis oil to break up bubbles.

Remove cannabis oil from heat when bubble formation starts to slow down — or leave on heat until all bubbles stop for increased sedative effect.

Table: Decarboxylation Temperatures and Times

Temperature +/- 5F	Heating Mode	Plant Material Time		Keif/Hash Time		Cannabis Oil Time
		High THC	*High CBD*	*High THC*	*High CBD*	
300F	Oven	10-18 minutes	15-25 minutes	5-10 minutes	10-15 minutes	
250F	Hot oil bath					Until bubbles taper off
245F	Oven	50-60 minutes	60 -90 minutes	30-40 minutes	40-50 minutes	
212F	Boiling water bath	90-120 minutes	2-4 hours	90-120 minutes	2-4 hours	

FACTS & FALLACIES

Some common misconceptions about cannabis has contributed to the demonization of an otherwise wonderful weed. Being informed is the easiest way to battle the beast of ignorance and aid in removing some of the archaic attitudes associated with cannabis. Therefore, since you've purchased this book and decided to learn more about bud let's remove a few fallacies -

YES. You are right and the rumors are true – POT is somewhat more potent today than it was in the 70's. WHY? What's changed in 40 years? First off, in the 1970s, note that most of the cannabis was imported. The potency of cannabis is affected by oxidation. Imports from outside of the country could take months to arrive, and during transport it was exposed to high temperatures, thus reducing the bud's potency. The popularization of hydroponics in the 80s led to spike in the potency in part because it was fresher but mostly the indoor growing revolution introduced cool new methods of cross breeding and hybridization creating many new strains. Better, more controlled growing conditions, ability to manipulate stock for desired genetics and in the 90's thanks to the internet, access to exponential amounts of information and resources - amateur farmers and professional breeders alike have changed the way we see weed!

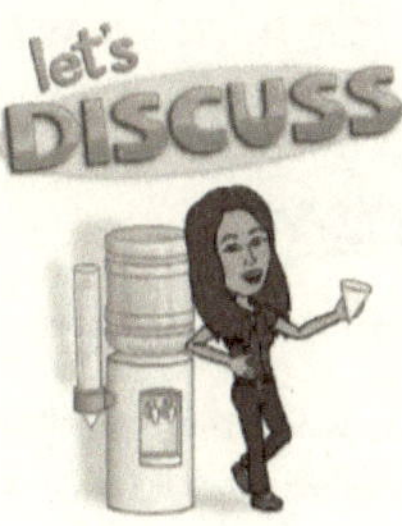

The next big question on the minds of many then is *"What's it like to be 'high'?"* and the easiest simplest answer is that it's a different experience for everyone for many reasons! From methods of consumption to selected strains and other influencing factors.

Anna Wilcox at Herb.co succinctly wrote– "In short, cannabis is quite different from alcohol in terms of effect. While all alcohol produces the same general effect, the cannabis experience varies significantly from person to person."
~Anna Wilcox – Herb.co

Whether you intend to utilize cannabis recreationally or medicinally, the **method of consumption can and will change the effect that the cannabinoids have on your brain & body.**

For the first-time consumer, the sensation of feeling "high" can be quite powerful. Giggle fits or yawn fests are not uncommon, and neither is an anxious or uneasy feeling. Experienced consumers will/do develop a tolerance to the cannabinoid THC –and for most cannabis fans the sensation of being high from herb is a pleasant, calm, relaxing bliss that lasts anywhere from 2 to 12 hours depending on the strain and method of consumption!

The high is nice, and quite frankly somewhat essential to a health and wellness strategy but realistically, there is so much more to cannabis than just the high.

In fact, there are entire health and wellness strategy programs built around the incorporation of cannabis into daily lifestyle - from diet and nutrition thru exercise and sleep – **FIGHT FIBRO GREEN & CLEAN** *created for Cannabis Corner Café* -is one such program that walks Fibromyalgia patients through a life changing 30-day program. More details are available on the website @ www.greenirene.ca Other cannabis infused programs include:

- **Learning to Live Again:** *Combining a combination of support tools, resources, and cannabis research, this program addresses the WHOLE person and takes a cannabis-infused holistic approach to health and wellness.*

- **Pain Management Strategies:** *Strategies for living a quality life **in spite of** chronic or complex pain. Enjoy your life right now – Incorporate cannabis as a tool or vehicle to help support your strategic plan of action – so that your life is lived, rather than "existing" or "getting through"*

Isn't every day a little too much? How much would cause a lethal overdose? These are very real concerns for the consumer who is considering cannabis use for the first time and or as part of their daily constituency. Even some somewhat seasoned consumers question the lethalness of cannabis –that being said understand that **No one ever in recorded history has died from a cannabis overdose - it is practically impossible to overdose.**

A hyperbolic media, crusading prohibitionists and a steady stream of drama driven do-gooders may have had you believing otherwise for many decades (I fell for the propaganda myself for many years – thankfully, INFO IS POWER)

https://www.youtube.com/watch?v=VMDWRvEJ5EA

In 1988 DEA brief, Judge Francis Young did the math and estimated that a smoker would theoretically have to consume nearly 1500 pounds of cannabis in about fifteen minutes or ingest approximately 22KG in one sitting to hypothetically induce a lethal response. A feat I suspect is rather improbable if not impossible, therefore, as you work with recipes RECOGNIZE that the measurements for cannabis can be modified without fear to find a dosage that is suitable for you.

Does all weed get you high? NO - not all cannabis is psychotropic (high inducing) *IN FACT, raw or still on the plant will not induce a psychotropic high at all.* TETRAHYDROCANNABINOL or THC (the cannabinoid that causes a high), like all the cannabinoids are produced and stored in the plant as ACIDS; THC-A does not become psychotropic until it is heated between 220 & 468 deg. F, converting it to THC - a process called DECARBOXYLATION.

Furthermore, because of hybridization/cross-breeding many plants have been bred to be high in CBD (not THC) and therefore offer little to no cerebral high.   Additionally, consumption methods - like applying a topical lotion or soaking in an infused bath will not produce any "high" as the cannabinoids are absorbed through the epidermal organ (skin) and do not break the blood/brain barrier.

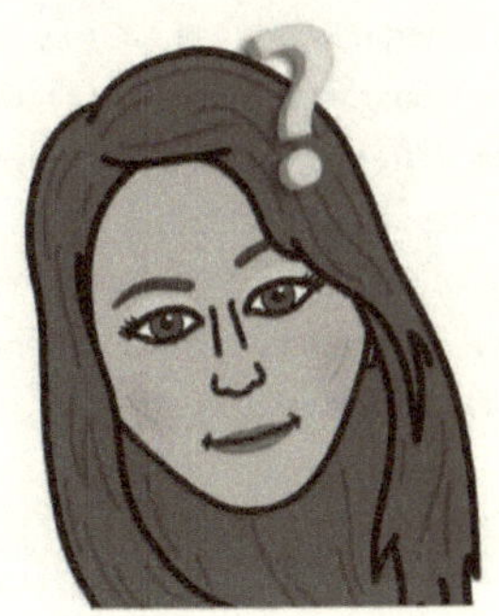

So, whether you are looking for the high or trying to avoid it - all things are possible and introducing cannabis into your life is easy. How you consume is as important to the overall effects, as is what you consume.

METHODS OR MEANS OF CONSUMPTION

The CURATIVE qualities of CANNABIS have been recognized by health and wellness practitioners for as long as recorded information has been obtainable - over 3000 years of documented information showing and proving the effectiveness of cannabis for treating ailments of the mind body and spirit – If you are ready to give it a try these are the most common methods of consumption and the overall general or expected effects.

Inhalation

There are three methods of inhalation that are frequently employed,

1. Smoking/Combustion,
2. Vaping, and/or
3. Dabbing.

Whenever breathed in, the cannabinoids are made effortlessly available to your brain and respiratory system. For this reason, inhaled cannabis tends to have a more immediate head-centered effect as compared to other consumption methods. The effects of inhaled cannabis can typically be felt within 5-10 minutes on average and the overall sensation can last 2 to 4 hours.

Combustion methods include rolling a joint, filling a bong bowl, smoking a pipe etc. Basically, the idea is to "burn" or combust the cannabis product in some way. This method of consumption is the most wasteful and ineffective way to truly enjoy and appreciate the product. Not to mention the least effective way to glean the value or benefit - medicinally and recreationally.

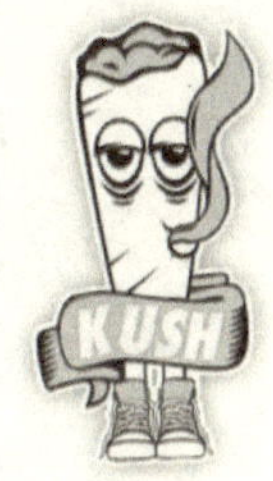

Why? Well as was stated earlier, THC is activated between 220°F & 468°F, heating the cannabis beyond that temperature essentially burns or boils most cannabinoids off. Because the cannabis plant produces more tar when burned than tobacco, the smoker is for all intent purposes consuming burnt plant material and tar- while the wonderfully rich cannabinoids evaporate into air and ash.

Carbon monoxide and tar are the 2 primary toxins released by combustion in the form of smoke. They are carcinogenic and can cause lung related problems. Others include Toleuene, Benzene and Maphthalene.

Vaporization.

This method of consumption is by far the best means of gleaning the most benefit from the cannabis plant. Complete and total control over temperatures allow for more accurate titration and an appreciation for pure flavour. Different cannabinoids, flavonoids and terpenes are released at different temperatures- using a digital vaporizing unit to heat the cannabis product provides the consumer with a significant amount of control over what is released from the plant material and when.

One of the advantages of vaporizers lies in their unique ability to extract the active ingredients of cannabis without the toxins of combustion. ***However, Vapor*** can still contain trace amounts of toxins. But one PAH

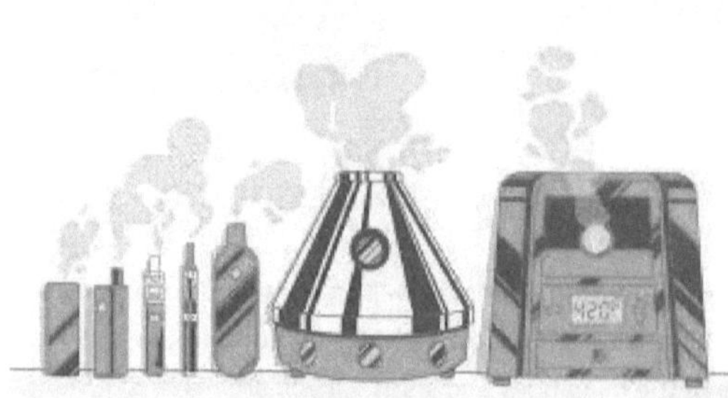

discovered in vapour is obviously a massive reduction compared to the over 100 different PAHs found in smoke. By the same token, toxins that come from pesticides, herbicides and other chemical agents can concentrate in the bud/flower and be released in vapour - that's why, growing your own, knowing your farmer or choosing organic cannabis is very wise and prudent choice.

The range of temperature in which all cannabinoids evaporate lies between 157 and 220 degrees Celsius (315 °F - 428 °F) .

A note about moisture

Bone dry cannabis can still be a delight in a vaporizer, unlike combusting it in a joint, bong or pipe. However, because it is so dry, it will vaporize much faster – if it is too hot you run the risk of flash boiling the active ingredients, eliminating taste and flavour. Lower the temperature for dry cannabis product there is no definitive temperature as it will vary according to strain and *how* dry it is.

Conversely, there can be significant moisture in fresh herb and the cannabinoids may not release easily. In this case, it is recommended to do what's called a flavonoid run. By putting the vaporizer at a lower temperature (around 138 – 148 °C or 280 °F - 298 °F.), it is possible to gain a bag of flavonoid vapour while at the same time, slowly drying out your herb. After this run, your cannabis should be dry enough to vaporize efficiently at temperatures suitable for THC and other desired cannabinoids.

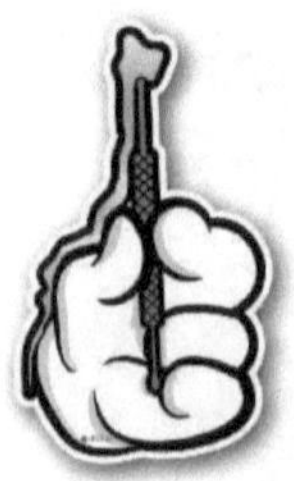

Dabbing:

Dabbing with cannabis concentrates is the biggest thing since the bong in the world of weed. They are concentrated doses of the cannabinoids extracted from the cannabis product - like THC and CBD.

Concentrates come as oils, wax, shatter, rosin, and probably a few other forms that I haven't heard of yet. Cannabis bud (flower/herb) typically contains 10-25% THC. By comparison, concentrates have closer to a range 75-95% THC thus offering/producing a monster high.

CBD concentrates are very effective therapeutically with little to no cerebral euphoria, but can be difficult to obtain as it's the THC hit that seems to have made the Concentrate Dabbing so popular among the recreational league of cannabis enthusiasts

Dabbing may seem daunting at first, but it's one of those activities that comes easily once you've seen it done. Essentially, dabbing is the flash vaporization of cannabis concentrates applied to a hot surface and inhaled. As you can imagine, these concentrates are a lot more potent than bud/herb, so a little bit goes a long way.

Dabbing isn't for everyone, especially the cannabis consuming newbie. The dosing process is delicate and takes some tolerance and patience to get the hang of - but once you do, concentrates can provide amazing physical relief and unique cerebral effects in very quick time with little product.

Sublingual Oils & Tinctures:

Sublingual is a complicated way to say, "taken under the tongue". The primary advantage is direct absorption into the bloodstream. Sublingual dropping is not only discreet it is a more palatable alternative for some medicinal users that require quick relief and for whatever reason cannot inhale or ingest.

This method of consumption is probably the least controversial because they are used primarily for medical treatment, not necessarily for recreation. Being they don't carry with them the fun association or time-honoured ceremony of …. passing the joint or sharing a balloon. Next to inhalation, sublingual tinctures produce the most immediate effects.

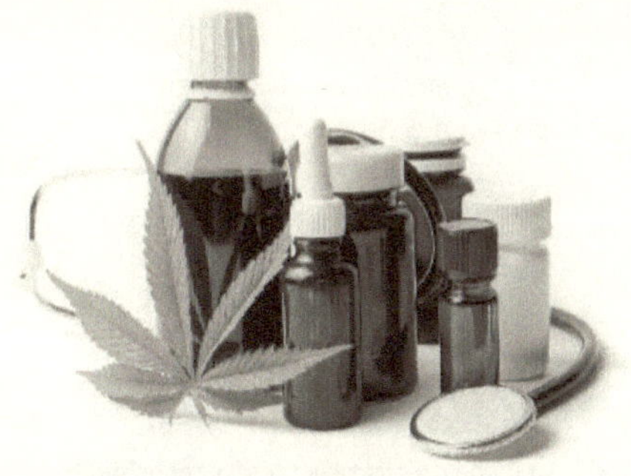

Through this method of administration, the cannabinoids immediately enter the bloodstream because the cavity under the tongue is filled with vessel-rich tissues. Sublingual dosing is the quickest form of relief; ideal for patients whose conditions require them to rely on fast-acting therapeutic effects. Sublingual application delivers the effects of cannabis in as little as 30 seconds.

More cannabis enthusiasts are discovering the benefits of sublingual delivery through cannabis oils and medicinal tinctures made of grain-alcohol or glycerine, akin to those of yesteryears pharmacopeia. Inhaling or ingesting is still the most popular means of consumption, but depending on your condition or desired intent, you may find it more effective to switch to sublingual dosing.

It is not difficult to imagine sublingual cannabinoid infused oils breaking into mainstream medicine and replacing a multitude of currently prescribed poisons. Alcohol based tinctures are also making a come back in the 'home remedy' kits and personal pharmacopeia journals. It's even easier to imagine high THC concentrate tinctures becoming sensationally popular.

Sublingual oils typically use a medium chain fat or triglyceride such as grape seed, palm kernel or sunflower oil etc., as a carrier for the cannabinoid admin; whereas, tincture recipes resemble the moonshine makers recipe book - try out a recipe or two for yourself!

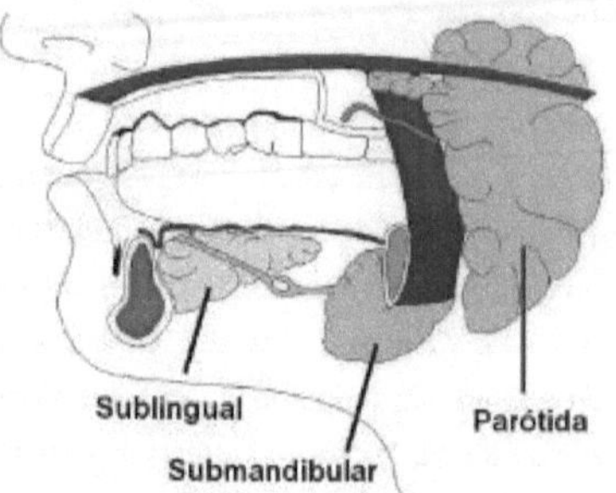

Aside from oils and tinctures, it's also completely possible to medicate by applying cannabis sublingually provided that it's already been decarboxylated. Using decarboxylated cannabis directly underneath the tongue can immediately deliver the cannabinoids into your bloodstream in the same way that tinctures and oils do but without the additional processing and product (oil/alcohol), which makes it healthier and more effective for many patients.

You won't achieve the same results or benefits if you use cannabis that hasn't been decarboxylated. This process is necessary to activate THCA into THC, which is a more powerful state of the cannabinoid. The use of heat through cooking (or smoking) is critical in the conversion of the cannabinoids.

The Basic Science of Tinctures

A tincture is most often an alcoholic extract of plant material (although animal material can also be used) with an ethanol percentage of between 25 and 60%. This equates to a solution that is between 50 and 120 proof, although sometimes the alcohol concentration can get as high as 90% (180 proof) in some tinctures.
~ Green Irene's **GUIDE TO CANNABIS TINCTURES**
www.greenirene.ca

Tincture recipes

The major advantage of this sublingual administration method is that the medicine is rapidly absorbed through the sublingual artery, which allows the medicine to quickly reach the brain. Additionally, the tincture doesn't come in contact with the acids in your stomach like other edibles do. That fact alone serves to keep many of the beneficial chemicals in your cannabis tincture more complete. You can, of course, swallow your tincture, or even add it to tea, juice or food like many patients do. Nothing bad will happen. However, the delta-9-THC in your tincture will transform into 11-Hydroxy-THC when it passes through the liver of your gastrointestinal tract. And depending on your metabolism, this can take up to two hours or more to occur. That means that you'll have to wait at least two hours to feel the effects.

It's also important to remember that you are also consuming alcohol—albeit a tiny amount—when you administer a tincture. In addition to that alcohol, your tincture will likely contain about 60% THC. That's a lot! **The combination of the alcohol and the THC can pack a hefty punch so start slow with your tincture titration**. Get a feel for the potency of your medication and then gradually increase your dosage. Err on the side of caution and start with 2 drops (or less) if you're new to cannabis consumption. After you administer your drops, wait at least an hour or so before consuming more. This gives the chemicals in the tincture time to spread throughout your body and gives your body time to fully process the cannabinoids.

Easy To Make

Tinctures are very economical and can be made by the do-it-yourself enthusiast rather easily. As mentioned, you can make marijuana tinctures out of grain alcohol or glycerin, but high-proof alcohol like Everclear is the most common solvent and is the easiest to use.

Tetrahydrocannabinol (THC), the active ingredient in all cannabis medication, exists as tetrahydrocannabinolic acid (THCA) until it is decarboxylated, usually with heat. The nice thing about the extraction process is that the alcohol bath dissolves the THCA, decarboxylates it into THC, and preserving the resultant material so that it doesn't spoil. The alcohol does all three of these things at the same time... without heat.

There are three basic methods for creating your own

- Cold
- Warm (a.k.a. Moonshine Marijuana)
- Hot (a.k.a. Green Dragon)

The Cold Method

The cold method is the easiest way to brew marijuana tinctures because it doesn't involve any cooking. All you have to do is mix the ingredients together and set it aside to brew. Here's how to do it.

- First, simply break your cannabis up into some smaller pieces and place it in a glass mason jar. You can use as much or as little marijuana as you like to strain into your tincture. Just make sure that the bud you use is dry. Fresh, moist weed just doesn't make for good tinctures.

- The next step is to pour in enough ethyl alcohol to keep the plant material covered. We suggest Everclear but you can use other high-proof alcohols if you prefer. You can expect to use approximately one gram of marijuana per one fluid ounce of ethyl alcohol. That said, the weed to alcohol ratio doesn't have to be exact. Just make sure the marijuana is covered.

- After you've mixed the ingredients in a jar, screw the lid on, shake it vigorously for a minute or two, then store the concoction in your freezer. The jar should stay there for up to 5 days. Don't worry, the jar won't break or shatter due to the expansion that occurs when liquids solidify. Alcohol has a much lower freezing point than water and will remain in the liquid state throughout this process.

- Once or twice a day for those 5 days, take the jar out of the freezer and give it a good shake. Over time, you'll see the plant matter start to dissolve.

- After roughly five days of storage in the freezer and multiple shakes every day, you've reached the end of the process. Now just strain the tincture through a cheesecloth, metal tea strainer, or silk screen into a bowl. Dispose of the leftover solid plant material and pour the liquid tincture into a small dark dropper bottle or two. It really is that simple!

The Warm Method - a.k.a. Moonshine method

It's called the MOONSHINE METHOD because the easiest way to may this one is '***to make it on the new moon; and strain on the full moon***'!

The warm or traditional method of making tinctures is identical to the cold method but without the freezer. Mix the ingredients in a mason jar the same as you did in the cold method. Then just leave the mason jar filled with weed and alcohol in a cool, dry place out of the sun for 30 to 60 days. After those 30 to 60 days have elapsed, separate the solid material from the liquid by straining and then distribute the tincture into dropper bottles. Yes, this method does take substantially longer than the cold method and the hot method, but it doesn't require any interaction on your part after the jar has been sealed.

The Hot Method - a.k.a. Green Dragon method

This is the quickest way to whip up a batch of cannabis tincture. It does require a bit of extra equipment and constant vigilance (so you don't set the alcohol on fire), but you'll reduce the brew time considerably.

- To begin, chop or grind the cannabis product as finely as you can. Place it on a cookie sheet in the oven at 325°F for about 5 minutes, or until your entire home begins to smell like weed. Mix your baked bud with high proof alcohol in a mason jar just like you did in the cold and warm methods.

- Place the opened mason jar in a pan and add about 1 inch of water around the mason jar. Don't put any water in the mason jar or you'll ruin your tincture. Bring the water to a boil and then simmer the uncovered mason jar until the temp reaches 165°F - use a thermometer. If the alcohol boils, the temperature is too high. Just turn down the heat of the water bath and continue. Additionally, it's usually a good idea to keep the kitchen fan on to remove any combustible alcohol fumes. At the very least, make sure that you are in a well-ventilated area so those fumes don't collect and ignite.

- When your brew has reached 165°F, remove the jar from the water bath using pot holders (it will be hot!), and set it aside to cool. When the jar is cool enough to handle with your bare hands, strain  the tincture into a glass container removing the plant matter from the liquid. Let the liquid cool some more and then distribute it into dropper bottles.

  Lastly, you can combine 5.5 grams of baked, decarboxylated cannabis with 2 ounces of high USP Food grade glycerine into a sealable mason jar and let it cook on top of a washcloth in a few inches of water in a crock pot on the low setting for 18-24 hours. Let the mixture cool for about 20 minutes then strain over a cheesecloth and use your dropper to transfer over to a tincture bottle.

Ingestion.

Cannabis in edible form has been a popular method of consumption since the 60s. The cannabinoids reach the cells by the way of the liver, which converts THC into another, more potent chemical, 11-hydroxy-THC. The digestion process affects the onset of euphoria, which takes approximately 30 to 60 minutes for the average person to feel. Which doesn't make it ideal for patients who need immediate or fast-acting relief. However, because the duration of effects lasts an average of 4-6 hours it is an excellent pain management tool for chronic pain sufferers who require long lasting effects.

Overconsumption or unusually high doses can result in effects lasting over 24 hours - so always use caution. The idea is LOW & SLOW to start. Furthermore, effects are more intense when consumed on an empty stomach and notably, alcohol increases the concentration of THC in the blood which heightens the intoxicating effects of cannabis.

Edibles can present in many forms, including baked goods, snacks, candy, ice cream, breads, juices and well... It can pretty much be infused into anything you eat or drink! So, depending on the purpose of your adventure, be it recreational or medicinal - anything is possible. A connoisseur is limited only by his or her imagination.

Cooking with cannabis is a super easy process – the titration and tolerance is the biggest challenge. SO LOW (dosage) & SLOW (wait 90 min between) - is always the motto! (Raw cannabis is the exception to that rule and more info follows.) That said, the 70s sensation of the good old pot brownies is passé! Today, one can find an exponential number of recipes that are cannabis infused. The internet hosts tons of explanatory videos and directions. Any food that appeals to your palate that can be prepared using oil or butter can easily be medicated and to really experiment with cooking, it is nice to have these infused items available.

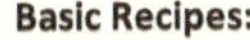

Basic Recipes:

● **Canna-Budder:** This recipe efficiently captures THC -CBD and other essential cannabinoids from your cannabis. It can be used as a straight substitution for anything that uses butter!

This is the easiest and best BASIC recipe.Here's what you'll need

**Ingredients**:

1 cup of water

1 lb. of butter, unsalted

1 oz. of high quality lightly ground cannabis bud, or trim (this amount equals very high potency - adjust accordingly)

**Equipment:**

Container with lid

Twine

Glass or ceramic bowl, refrigerator and heat safe

Pot

Stove

Spatula

Knife

Cheese cloth

Baking sheet or oven pan

Step 1. Decarboxylate bud

Preheat oven to 215 degrees Fahrenheit or 102 degrees Celsius. Break the flowers (bud) into small pieces. Spread evenly over the surface of the pan and cover with aluminum foil. Bake for 30 minutes.The cannabis will be light brown, dried out, and the active ingredients will be more concentrated.

Step 2. Add butter and water to stove pot, cook on low, throw in the weed

Add butter and water to cooking pot and simmer on low. The water will prevent the butter from burning. As the butter melts, add decarbed ground cannabis.

Step 3. Simmer 3 hours

Keep the mixture simmering on low for 3-4 hours stirring occasionally. Make sure it doesn't reach a boil. Then remove from heat and let it cool enough to safely touch.

Step 4. Strain out plant material with cheesecloth

Tie your cheesecloth with twine to make a lid covering your glass or ceramic bowl or other container. Carefully pour the hot mixture into your bowl while straining it with the cheese cloth to remove all plant substance. You can also use a permanent coffee filter or mesh for straining.

Tip/idea: Consider wrapping the cannabis product in cheesecloth before adding it to oil or butter for infusion. The discovery that potency is not lost by wrapping up the weed has become a major time saver for many!

Step 5. Refrigerate for hardening

Remove the cheesecloth. Cover the mixture and place it in the refrigerator for hardening. The butter will separate from the water and you will remove it with your spatula or other tool and place it in a storage container for use. Dispose of the remaining water.

Dosing: Divide into 28 pieces

Now it is time to enjoy your canna-budder! Dosing doesn't have to be overly tricky. Titration, for most is the biggest challenge, so this simple tip may be helpful.

Since the recipe calls for one ounce of decarboxylated cannabis, theoretically dividing the butter into 28 equal pieces - each piece yields the equivalent of approximately 1gram of weed. The rule is "start low and go slow" for cannabis edibles. Wait 90 minutes before redosing.

Recipe: Canna-Oil

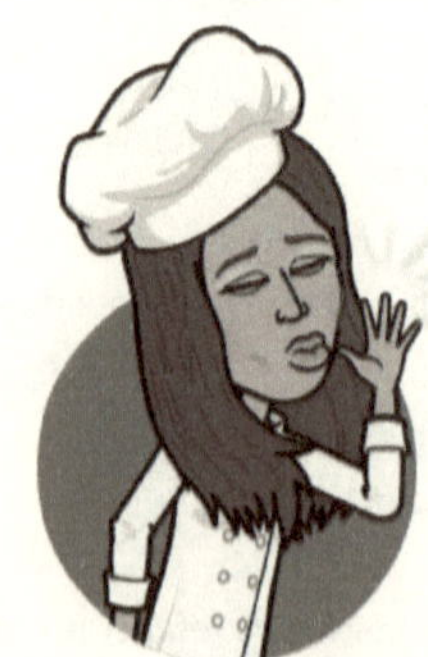

- Cannabis infused cooking oils, commonly referred to as canna oils, are popular for use in everything from salad dressings to dipping sauces to baked goods. Most oils are vegan-friendly and extremely easy to add into recipes with savory meals like steak or chicken.

Additionally, infused cooking oils may serve as a healthy substitute for butter in many recipes. These factors make canna-infused cooking oils a must-have for most when it comes to cooking with cannabis at home.!

Ingredients:

- 6 cups extra virgin olive oil (organic preferred) (or)canola oil (backup oil — not preferred)
- 1 ounce cannabis buds, finely ground (or) ~2 ounces of leaf trim, dried and finely ground

INSTRUCTIONS:

- In a heavy saucepan (or a double boiler), slowly heat the cooking oil on low heat for a few minutes. You should begin to smell the aroma coming from the oil.
- Add a little bit of cannabis to the oil and then stir until it is fully coated with oil. Keep adding more cannabis until the entire amount of cannabis is mixed into the oil.
- Simmer on low heat for 45-50 minutes, stirring occasionally.
- Remove the mixture from the heat and allow it to cool before straining.
- Press the cannabis against a metal strainer with the back of a spoon to wring all the oil out of it.
- The oil is best stored in an airtight container in the refrigerator for up to 2 months.
- Throw the leftover cannabis in the compost.

Infusion Suggestions

Any affordable virgin olive oil works nicely for this recipe. If you plan on using your cannabis cooking oil for salad dressings or pasta, it is recommended that you use a fruity EVOO to enhance the flavors.

Using raw cannabis

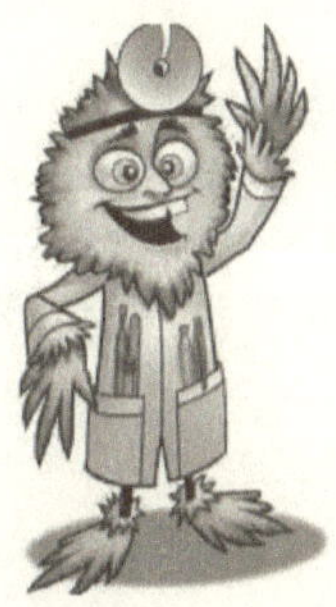

Raw cannabis is not psychoactive, meaning that you won't/can't get high! For all intent purposes, its akin to eating grapes hoping to get drunk!!! Raw cannabis will NOT induce a euphoria (high). To get the full psychoactive effect, the plant matter needs to be activated through the process of decarboxylation. However, there are several surprisingly good reasons - some claim that cannabis **is** the **new superfood** and should be added to our diet as part of a health and wellness strategy plan.

Raw cannabis is nutrient-dense powerhouse, having a big nutritional impact even in small doses. If you're skeptical, here are a few facts to consider.:

Protein: 30 grams (2 tablespoons) of shelled hemp seed contains 11 grams of protein. As far as plants are concerned, this is a rarity. Even the power-packed chia seed falls behind hemp in terms of overall protein per serving.

In contrast, chia seed contains about 4 grams per serving. This makes hemp a particularly valuable protein source for vegans and vegetarians.

Cannabinoid Acids: Preclinical research suggests that THCA potentially has antiproliferative and antispasmodic effects. The acid has also been found to trigger a certain cell receptor called TRPA1, which plays an important role in pain regulation and inflammation related to the nervous system.

The raw, acid form of cannabidiol (CBD), a cannabinoid that is being researched as a potential new treatment for epilepsy, also has shown some potential. Early research has shown that CBDA connects with the same cell receptors as some over the counter anti-inflammatory drugs. CBDA also interacts with the TRPA1 receptor, giving it some pain-fighting potential. **VISIT AND WATCH:** https://youtu.be/IlsBGXNxJYU

Courtney also articulates that the standard dose of raw cannabis can be significantly higher than a dose of

---

According to Dr. William Courtney, a doctor that recommends raw cannabis to patients, cannabinoid acids are,

    a.   Anti-inflammatory

    b.   Antioxidant

    c.   Anti-diabetic

    d.   Anti-ischemic

    e.   Have anti-tumoural effects

---

activated cannabis. While the recommended dose of activated THC is about 10 oral milligrams, a dose of raw cannabis acids can be up to a thousand milligrams.

- **Fibre**: Consuming high-fiber foods is needed to maintain proper digestion and to cultivate a healthy microbial community in your digestive tract.
  Fiber is broken down by microbes that live in the intestines. These microbes are essential for human survival, and recent research shows that caring for this internal ecosystem is vital for proper immune function and mental health. To keep these microorganisms alive and in balance, eating fibrous foods is key. Cannabis, is just like other leafy green and is high in fibre and can be used in

salads dishes, on sandwiches and in smoothies - just to name a few creative ways to incorporate it into one's menu plan.

- **Vitamins**: Like other green leafy plants, cannabis fan leaves contain a variety of vitamins and minerals. Leafy greens are filled with nutrients like:
    i. Folate (essential for DNA repair)
    ii. Iron (essential for moving oxygen through the blood)
    iii. Calcium (essential for strong bones)
    iv. Vitamin C (essential for immune function)
    v. Vitamin K (essential for blood clotting and calcium absorption)
    vi. Cannabis is special and also contains cannabinoid acids.

ALL edible dark leafy greens contain compounds that protect against cancer development. All in all, the greater the variety of greens, the better.

- **Hemp seeds** are a good source of a few different vitamins and minerals. The first is vitamin E. Vitamin E is a fat-soluble antioxidant that helps maintain healthy skin, hair, and immune function. Two tablespoons of hemp seed contain up to 77% of the daily value of vitamin E. 30 grams (2 tablespoons) of shelled hemp seed contains over 48% of your daily value of magnesium, which is necessary for over 300 biochemical reactions in the body. Unfortunately, at least half of Americans are deficient in this vital mineral.

- **Antioxidants:** Cannabinoids like CBD and THC are considered antioxidants, meaning that they protect the body from damage from stress. Raw cannabis also contains antioxidants, making it a great way to get a healthy boost of anti-aging nutrients without experiencing a psychoactive high.

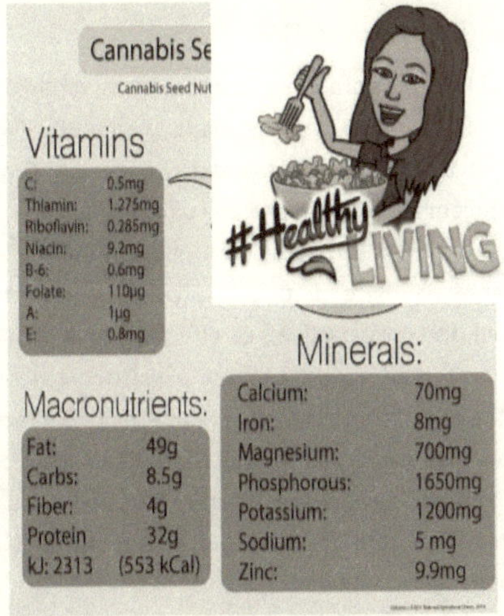

- **Anthocyanins:** Have some purple cannabis leaves? Eat them! Deep red, purple, and blue coloration in cannabis means that the plant is filled with flavonoid compounds called anthocyanins. Anthocyanins give the rich color to foods like blackberries, black tomatoes, plums, eggplant, and red raspberries.

Research shows that anthocyanins have a protective effect on human health. A 2004 review suggests that these colorful compounds are antioxidants themselves, protecting against DNA damage. They also seem to provide protection against hormone-dependent diseases, regulate the immune response, and some may even help improve vision in concentrated doses.

- **Essential fatty acids**

Eating enough fatty acids is essential for a healthy endocannabinoid system (ECS). Fortunately, hemp seed contains an awful lot of fatty acids. In fact, a tablespoon of hemp seed can contain up to 1000 mg of omega-3 fatty acids, and 2500 mg of omega-6 fatty acids.

Omega fatty acids are essential for brain health, and many neurological and mental health conditions are associated with inadequate omega-3 intake. Hemp is also a great source of gamma linolic acid (GLA), which is a type of omega 6 fatty acid with unique characteristics.

While many omega 6 fatty acids are thought to promote inflammation, GLA appears to have the opposite effect. GLA has a wealth of potential health benefits, including:

- Easing diabetic neuropathy
- Easing arthritis pain
- Managing acne
- Managing eczema
- Easing symptoms of ADD/ADHD

The bottom line… raw cannabis is a lovely and flavourful way to get into a diet that is "Green & Clean" One of the greatest uses of the cannabis plant is actually through the nutrition it provides. Raw cannabis will likely become a staple source of nutrition in the years to come as the persecution and ignorance of this amazing plant is washed away.

There are a number of great cannabis-infused recipe cookbooks available through amazon and at Cannabis Corner Cafe Vape Lounge & Info Center in Penetanguishene ON or via www.cannabiscornercafe.ca

Topical solutions

Cannabis topicals are products like creams, lotions, salves and oils made for external use. They can be made with CBD, THC, or THCA (the non-psychoactive cannabinoid found in raw plants). They are most often used to treat inflammation, pain and skin conditions.

They are a great introduction for people entering into the holistic world of cannabis. As these ointments provide a powerful dose of medication 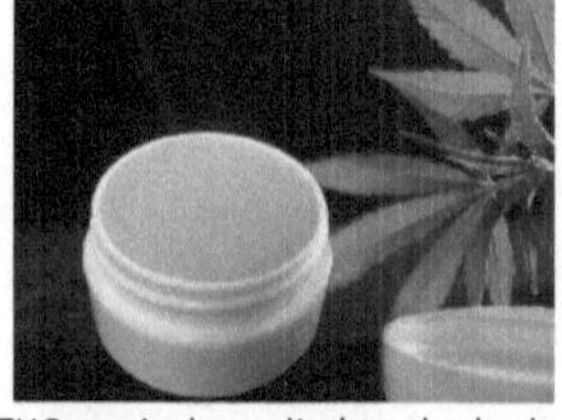 without the psychoactive side effects. Even with high levels of pain-fighting THC, topicals applied to the body do not enter the bloodstream and so will not present in standard drug testing. The cannabinoids when absorbed into the epidermis bind to the endocannabinoid receptors in the skin providing localized pain relief.

As identified earlier, our bodies contain two main cannabinoid receptors: CB1, the psychoactive receptor that also mediates pain and many other functions, and CB2, a non-psychoactive receptor that mediates pain and inflammation both are operative in the skin and affect pain, itch and inflammation associated with many dermatological conditions.

Despite being one of the safest and easiest methods of using cannabis, topicals are also one of the lesser known and under-utilized. However, they are gaining in popularity INFO IS POWER. Common stigmas against cannabis tend to dissolve minds of skeptics when they find such positive and unique relief from cannabis infused topical products without any of the negative side effects that are unfairly attached to marijuana. Topical cannabis ointments are great at providing relief to people with conditions like arthritis or chronic back pain., and for good reason. Topicals are incredibly easy to use.It's as simple as rubbing a product onto any area experiencing pain or discomfort, including sore muscles post-workout, itchiness from skin conditions such as eczema or even joint pain from arthritis.

Different forms of cannabis topicals have been used throughout history. In early Indian medicine, for instance, cannabis was mixed with other ingredients to make a surgical anesthetic. Other ancient examples include a Tibetan treatment for itchy skin and traditional Arabic remedies for skin ailments and hair growth.

That being said …. you can make your own quite affordably.

Making CannaBalm

Similar to making CannaButter, CannaBalm requires a fatty base – but this time it should be a base that can be stored at room temperature for several weeks. Coconut oil and shea butter are the most common choices for creams and ointments, but some people prefer the extra body offered by the harder beeswax, which can be used as the sole base or added in varying proportions depending on the desired result. Lip balm, for example, would use a larger proportion of edible-grade beeswax.

Almond and grapeseed oil are sometimes added (as a percentage of the overall base material) to enhance penetration of the balm, and aloe vera is an additive believed to add antibacterial activities. Make sure that if you add these ingredients, you subtract the same amount from the total volume of your base. In other words, if you are adding 2 TBL of almond oil, subtract 2 TBL from the recipe's cup of coconut oil.

Equipment

Grinder

CookieSheet

Aluminum Foil

Heavy, medium-size double boiler (Two pans, one slightly smaller than the other, that can function as a double boiler)

Water (for bottom of double boiler)

Candy Thermometer

Spoon or Spatula

Fine mesh strainer/sieve

Heatproof Glass Bowl (for strained balm)

Storage Container

Ingredients

1 Cup of Coconut Oil, Beeswax or Shea Butter (or a combination)

1 Ounce Ground Cannabis Bud

Directions

Finely grind the cannabis bud and decarboxylate (See Decarboxylate) it for maximum potency. To do this, spread your ground cannabis on a cookie sheet, cover with tinfoil and bake at 230°F for 45 minutes.

Place the water-filled bottom of the double boiler over medium heat. Add your base to the top pan. Use a candy thermometer to make sure your base temperature doesn't exceed 240 degrees. Add your decarboxylated marijuana. Simmer, stirring occasionally, for at least 30 minutes.

Fit the strainer over the glass bowl. Strain the marijuana mixture into the bowl, allowing it to drain completely

through the strainer. Cool for about an hour, then transfer the cannabalm to a clean container and store for about two weeks. If you use a mixture of oils, they may separate over time. Gently reheat to reconsititute.

Thankfully, the normalization of cannabis use is changing the market and product development opportunities are limited only by creativity! Currently the market is expanding exponentially. An industry leader, Doc Green's is joined by popular brands including Colorado's Mary's Medicinals, which is best known for its transdermal patches and transdermal gel pens.. Other popular brands include_Whoopi Goldberg's line of products aimed at relieving menstrual pain, and Mary Jane's Medicinals to name a few.

WHY use Cannabis?

Cannabis users are often portrayed as unmotivated, lazy "stoners", hippy hang-overs, pot heads and dead heads." However, INFO IS POWER and research into why people use cannabis paints an entirely different picture than that of a media influenced stigma. It shows that most people use cannabis as a rational choice to enhance the quality of their life. Cannabis affects people in different ways. It's effects are dependant on many factors including the person, the situation, the strain and quality of cannabis, as well as the method of consumption. Research shows that most people who use cannabis use it moderately and have been doing so for thousands of years - for social, medical and spiritual reasons. Often the reasons for consumption overlap.

Social Use

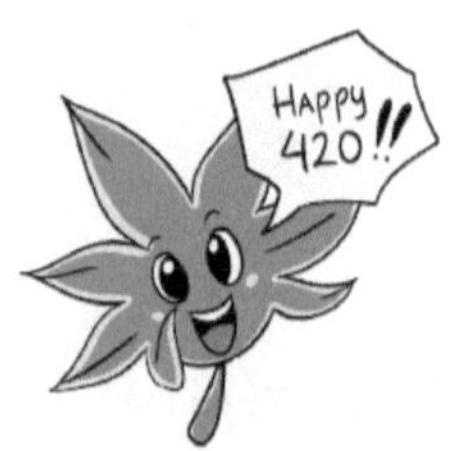

The social use of cannabis includes its consumption for recreation, socializing and generally improving quality of life. As cannabis becomes *"normalized"* (through legalization and education) "Bud over Booze" is a choice made by many for good reasons, but mostly because it is a less damaging intoxicant than alcohol - mentally, physically, emotionally, socially, financially and spiritually!
In fact many would argue that it is NOT a damaging intoxicant at all. Cannabis is a cure - Mind, Body & Soul.

There are many historical references made to the social use of cannabis. Ancient Hindus in India were against the use of alcohol, but openly accepted social cannabis consumption. In ancient Rome, the affluent or wealthy would wrap up banquets by serving a cannabis-seed dessert that was known to induce euphoria. At ancient Indian weddings cannabis in the drink form known as bhang was served for good luck and as a sign of hospitality, much in the same way we serve wine!
Social use of cannabis often becomes part of a person's daily routine without negative consequences to their health, social, legal or economic conditions. In fact, most who use it daily find it improves the quality of their lives. As it helps some to relax and concentrate making many activities more pleasant and enjoyable such as

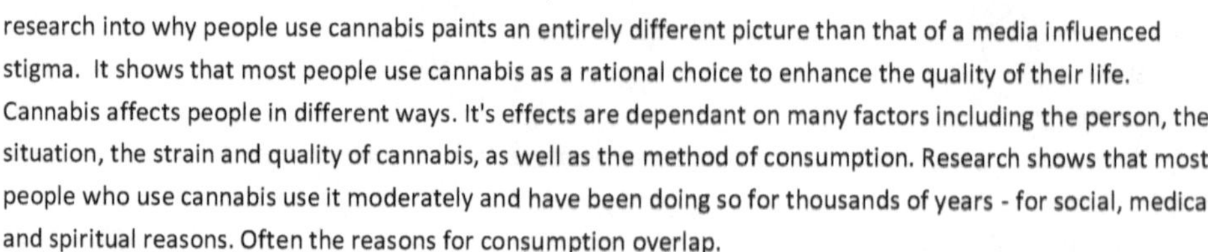

eating, listening to music, socializing, watching movies and being creative to name a few. Some people even claim they use it to make mundane chores tolerable!

The World Health Organization Constitution defines health as "a state of complete physical, mental and social well-being, and not merely the absence of disease or infirmity." Therefore, the social uses of cannabis sometimes coincide with, or complement, its medical uses.

Medical Use

Like people who use cannabis for social reasons, people who use cannabis for medical reasons also use it to

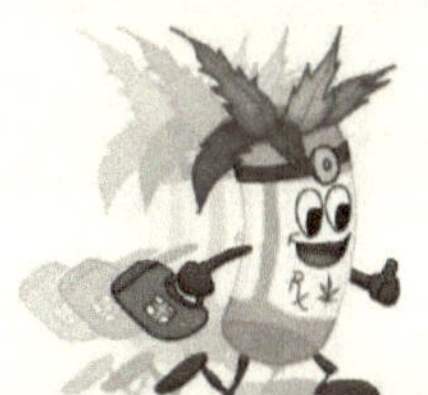

improve their quality of life. Medical use is linked to managing physical and mental problems and to preserving health.

Cannabis has been used medically for thousands of years. In 2700 BCE, Shen Neng, Chinese Emperor and father of Chinese medicine, used cannabis as a remedy. The Ebers Papyrus, an ancient Egyptian medical text, also mentions cannabis. It was written in 1500 BCE and is one of the oldest pharmaceutical works known.

In Canada, cannabis was used as a medicine until it was added to a list of controlled substances in 1923 - for the record, no one really knows why or how it got introduced or added, there certainly wasn't a vote on the subject!   Anyway, in 2000, patients won the right to again use cannabis legally as a medicine. The court ruled that people should not have to choose between their liberty and their health because both are protected in the constitution.

Cannabis is used to treat many medical conditions and symptoms. It is effective in treating nausea, loss of appetite, pain, anxiety, insomnia, inflammation and muscle spasms. These symptoms are often part of physical or mental conditions. Arthritis, cancer, HIV/AIDS, multiple sclerosis, epilepsy, Parkinson's disease, ADHD and post-traumatic stress disorder are some conditions cannabis can help treat.

Pharmaceuticals or not – pills or pot BIG question on the minds of many. Be empowered by education, not fueled by opinion. Do your research and become the FIRST line of defense in your health and wellness strategy.

Physical energy must be mastered and grounded for spiritual energy to move, because physical energy transforms the spirit.

–Teilhard de Chardin

Spiritual Use

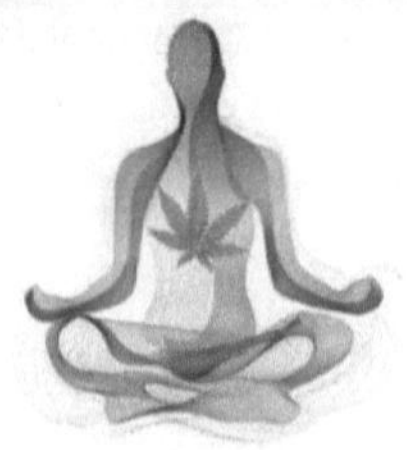

Spiritual well-being is widely accepted as an important part of overall health. Spiritual use of cannabis relates to seeking a sense of meaning, enlightenment and connection.

Some claim that the great visionaries packed sacred pipes with cannabis because smoking increased the intensity of their visions. Cannabis has a rich history of spiritual use. It is listed as one of the five holy plants in the Atharvaveda, a sacred Indian text from the second millennium BCE. The Scythians, who lived in what is now Eastern Europe, used cannabis at funerals to pay respect to departed leaders. Ancient Chinese texts say that cannabis can lighten a person's body and allow them to communicate with spirits. The Persian prophet Zoroaster (7 BCE) relied on the intoxicating effects of bhanga, a cannabis drink, to bridge heaven and earth. Some researchers believe that kannabosm, a plant mentioned in the Old Testament as an ingredient in the sacred anointing oil, was an ancient name for cannabis.

Today, some people use cannabis in their spiritual practice. Rastafarians and some Hindus and Sikhs continue to use cannabis in religious ceremonies. Modern spiritual figures like Ram Dass openly acknowledge that the use of cannabis has allowed them to gain a more spiritual perspective and use the herb frequently for both its medicinal and mind-altering properties. In Mexico, followers of the Santa Muerte regularly use marijuana smoke in purification ceremonies, with marijuana often taking the place of incense used in otherwise mainstream Catholic rituals.

Other people use it in ways they consider spiritual, such as for reflection, contemplation or personal growth. The relaxing effects of cannabis help some people gain a different perspective when trying to understand difficult life situations and so is often employed prior or during a meditation practice. Some believe that cannabis, as a plant, has something to teach them.

Cannabis is used by some to increase an appreciation for and connection with nature and frequently paired with Yoga practices. People also use cannabis to bond with each other as can be seen by social group gatherings. These feelings of connectedness contribute to an overall sense of "oneness." that is essential to harmonious health and wellness.

GROW YOUR OWN

There hasn't been a better time than now to become a cannabis cultivator - with or without a green thumb - You can do it! The benefits of growing your own are multi-fold, but the main reasons are:

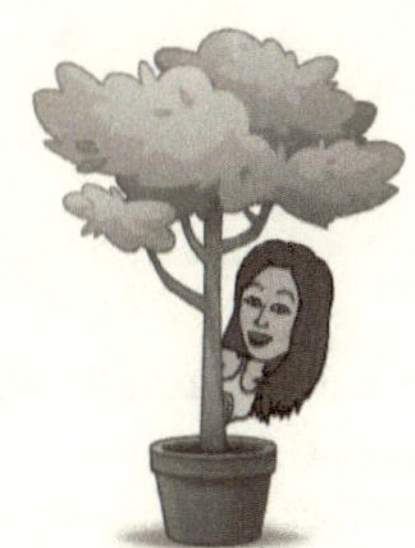

1. **TO SAVE MONEY** - growing your own bud has a huge cash saving component, you'll be surprised at just how much. Whether you use cannabis medicinally or recreationally, growing a few plants will provide you with a steady flow of weed so you won't need to buy it at $7-$15 a gram.

Sure, some growers end up spending some extra money on materials and equipment, but that initial investment will soon pay off. Alternatively, to really drive down costs, some decent seeds and a good amount of rich soil is all that is truly required.

Second only to the cash savings is the confidence that you know exactly what you're getting. Both recreational and medicinal cannabis users place a lot of importance on the quality of the products they're using. By growing your own, you can say goodbye to the worries of *how* your weed was grown, *what* fertilizers it was given, *whether* it was flushed/cured correctly, etc.

Homegrown has come a long way since the days of total prohibition... Are you ready to start growing?

There is plenty of reliable information available on the internet that can teach cannabis users exactly how to grow and process weed correctly in the comfort of their own home. However, before you flex that green thumb of yours, understand that the sheer volume of information available on the subject can be overwhelming. Every budtender, farmer and hobbyist have an opinion and as such is not necessarily based on fact or knowledge but rather "Trial and error". The secret therefor is quite simply... "start with what you know and grow with the flow" it's a process of experimentation and a labor of love.

A lot of people unintentionally make growing harder than it needs to be - perhaps because it's a wonder weed - but it really is just a weed and growing the cannabis plant is pretty straightforward. Basically, anyone with a few extra minutes a day and a spare closet or a garden in the back yard can grow their own private stock at home.

One of the most common mistakes by new cannabis growers is conducting spur-of-the-moment experiments that hurt or possibly even kill their plants. Always take a second to google your idea before you try it. Luckily when it comes to growing cannabis, chances are someone has tried it already!

TAKE RESPONSIBILITY FOR THE QUALITY OF YOUR LIFE – GROW YOUR OWN FOOD & MEDICINE:

Many of the original cultures and people knew and understood that GOOD HEALTH meant more than just physical healing. For healing to truly be successful the physical, mental, emotional and spiritual had to be addressed. In our ego-centric driven healthcare system, mainstream western science rules and focuses primarily on the functions of the physical. A fascinating study – absolutely, but not enough knowledge or care for true and complete healthcare or healing.

There's an old, old saying that it's the spirit plus the person plus the medicine plus the healer that equals holistic health.

Native teachings, as I have come to understand them within my own cultural reference (Anishinaabe/Ojibwe) continue to have significant influence along this healing journey. A quick comparison of values….

Traditional Native Medicine: The primary focus takes an integrated, holistic approach to health; attention is given to the physical, emotional, intellectual and spiritual so that all aspects of the human condition can heal in synchronicity.

Significant emphasis is put on the prevention of disease. Each person is responsible for their own health and wellness, though there is significant guidance and support from peers and elders, as well as healers of Midewiwin . Health and sickness are considered and understood in accordance with the terms of the laws of nature. Traditional medicine is governed by the laws of creation: everything we need comes from earth – our food, medicines, water, education, spirituality and laws. The medicine man or woman is accountable to the creator, the people, and to

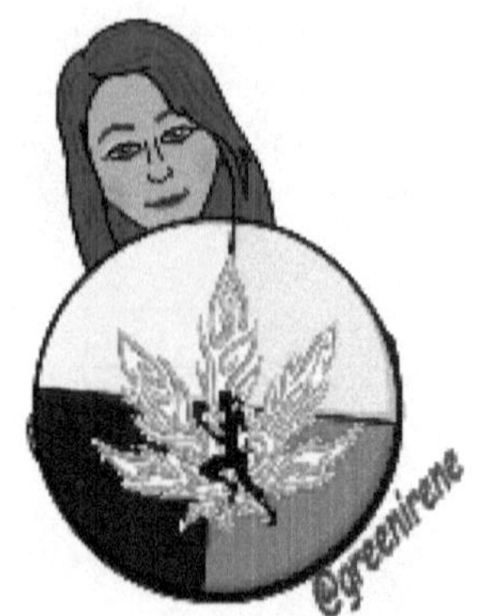

the elders of the medicine society (Midewiwin). Medicine is not for sale, not for profit – it is a gift to be shared, because of this the land and the people support the medicine man/woman and his practice. Traditional native medicine encourages self-sufficiency, self-care and responsibility.

Western medicine by contrast takes an analytical approach; separation of body mind emotion and spirit. The emphasis is on disease and understood in terms of quantifiable scientific data. It is an impersonal scientific approach to health, sickness and treatment. Furthermore, western medicine is governed by laws of the state, man-made laws growing out of political-economic systems. Medicine is BIG BUSINESS, with good return on investment. The western medicine system encourages dependency and abdication of self-government by the people.

It's your life – your body – your future and the mark you'll make while you're alive is all yours. Take control and do something today that you'll thank yourself for tomorrow.
INFORMATION IS POWER

Books, magazines, websites, forums, online and in-person growing communities—these are just a few examples of ways in which growers are sharing the bounty of their knowledge. Long gone are the days of whispering or hiding what you know.

The internet is host to multiple weekly podcasts dedicated to cannabis cultivation, an exponential number of "how to" YouTube videos and a host of websites/blogs dedicated to the subject. These are not only exciting times for cannabis enthusiasts everywhere, but the perfect time for the new home grower to get started!

CONCLUSION

Having a greater understanding of WHAT cannabis is, HOW it's grown and utilized as well as WHY it is consumed aids in removing the archaic attitude attached to this wonderful weed. The incredible curative powers of cannabis - mind, body & spirit, have been hidden in the closet for nearly a century - but no more!

FEAR IS DEBILITATING:

INFORMATION IS POWER.

Green Irene is available as a guest or keynote speaker. Very well versed about cannabis and the numerous subtopics. Available by the hour, half day or full days for seminars, workshops and event presentations.

BOOK A MEET & GREET NOW TO DETERMINE HOW I CAN EMPOWER YOUR GROUP/AUDIENCE

PRESENTATIONS INCLUDE BUT NOT LIMITED TO:

- **BUD BASICS:** *Cannabis 101, covering all the basic FAQs related.*
- **ATTACK ARTHRITIS:** *Incorporating cannabis as a strategy for symptom relief – how and why it works.*
- **BATTLE BEASTLY BOWELS:** *The cannabis connection to the digestive system.*

- ■ **PILLS or POT**: *Medical considerations, therapeutic strategies and what this plant is not.*
- ■ **From Leaf to Law with Logic:** *Understanding the evolution of the nascent industry. Curing curiosities, filling in the blanks of missing information and clearing up some mis-info surrounding the subject of cannabis and it's consumption.*
- ■ **FIGHT FIBROMYALGIA**: *Green and Clean patients can manage fibromyalgia fatigue, flare-ups, fog and more. Learn to use the leaf to your advantage and regain the quality of life you deserve.*
- ■ **STRAINS FOR PAINS:** *A unique summary, analysis, and explanation of what to use when and how. From phenotypes to methods of consumption this presentation covers it all, empowering chronic pain sufferers.*
- ■ **AND MORE…** *The curiosities surrounding cannabis and its consumption, acquisition, and legalities as a product, therapy, industry or nutritional supplement are as plentiful as there are stars in the night sky.*
- ■ **HAVE A TOPIC YOU'D LIKE TO HAVE ME SPEAK ON?** *Let's do a "MEET & GREET" to see if I'm the right speaker/presenter for your audience.* **CLICK HERE TO SCHEDULE**

Considering CANNABIS as a…

Medicinal treatment? Therapeutic strategy? Nutritional supplement?
I offer **consultations**, **guidance**, **assistance**, **information** and more –

GREEN IRENE'S CANNABIS SUPPORT CLINIC

*Offers information-packed, powerful coaching sessions designed to **EMPOWER YOU** to become the first line of defense, taking control over the quality of your life through a cannabis-infused health and wellness strategy plan.*

• *__You will gain__ a greater understanding of Cannabis, the medicinal and nutritional benefits that can be gleaned from different methods of consumption and how that applies to you. The skills for infusing your diet and exercise programs, as well as a favorable level of competency for titrating and managing cannabis consumption.*

As we move through our coaching work together, you'll find yourself more able to translate all the info you've gathered into the do-able steps and strategies that work for you – to live life again in spite of chronic conditions and manage the quality of your health and wellness effectively

This publication is authored by Irene A York as the first book of the INFO IS POWER

SERIES produced for Cannabis Corner Café by GREENIRENE

www.greenirene.ca

PRE-ORDER FUTURE TITLES INCLUDE:

1. **Bud Basics**
2. **Sleep Solutions – Bud for bedtime**
3. **Attack Arthritis**
4. **M.A.D. Cannabis – Mood, Anxiety & Depression**
5. **Bowel Battles – Get on the pot and poop!**
6. **Migraine Management with Mari-jane**
7. **PTSD, OSI & PTSI – The cannabis solution**
8. **Medical management**

... and several other Topic titles in turn!

Resources used for compiling the information

contained in BUD BASICS part INFO IS POWER SERIES produced for Cannabis Corner Café, authored by Irene A York (a.k.a Green Irene):

1. Osborne, G.B. and Fogel, C. (2008). Understanding the motivations for recreational marijuana use among adult Canadians. *Substance Use & Misuse*, 43(3), 539-572.

2. Hathaway, A. (2003). Cannabis effects and dependency concerns in long-term frequent users: A missing piece of the public health puzzle. *Addictions Research and Theory*, 11(6): 441-458.

3. Looby, A. & Earlywine, M. (2007). Negative consequences associated with dependence in daily cannabis users. *Substance Abuse Treatment, Prevention, and Policy, 2(3)*.

4. Melamede, R. (2005). Harm reduction—The cannabis paradox. *Harm Reduction Journal*, 2(17). www.harmreductionjournal.com/content/2/1/17.

5. Nutt, D., King, L.A., Saulsbury, W. et al. (2007). Development of a rational scale to assess the harm of drugs of potential misuse. *The Lancet,* 369(9566): 1047-1053.

6. Russo, E.B. (2007). History of cannabis and its preparations in saga, science, and sobriquet. *Chemistry and Biodiversity*, 4(8), 1614-1648.

7. Thomas, G., Flight., J., Richard, K. et al. (2006). *Toward a policy-relevant typology of cannabis use for Canada: Analysis drawn from the 2004 Canadian Addiction Survey*. Ottawa: Canadian Centre for Substance Abuse. www.ccsa.ca/2006%20CCSA%20Documents/ccsa-011334-2006.pdf.

8. Hanus, L.O. (2008). Pharmacological and therapeutic secrets of plant and brain (endo)cannabinoids. *Medicinal Research Reviews*, 29(2), 213-271.

9. Le Dain Commission. (1972). *Cannabis: A report of the Commission of Inquiry into the Non-Medical Use of Drugs*. Ottawa: Information Canada.

10. Government of Canada. (2001, July). Marihuana Medical Access Regulations. *Canada Gazette* (Part II), 135(14). www.gazette.gc.ca/archives/p2/2001/2001-07-04/pdf/g2-13514.pdf.

11. Canadian Centre on Substance Abuse. (2004). *Canadian addiction survey 2004*. Ottawa: Author. www.ccsa.ca/eng/priorities/research/CanadianAddiction/Pages/default.aspx.

12. Stockwell, T., Sturge, J., Jones, W. et al. (2007). *Cannabis use in British Columbia: Patterns of use, perceptions and public opinion as assessed in the 2004 Canadian Addictions Survey*. Centre for Addictions Research of BC, University of Victoria, and Centre for Applied Research on Mental Health and Addictions, Simon Fraser University. carbc.ca.

13. Preamble to the Constitution of the World Health Organization as adopted by the International Health Conference, New York, 19-22 June 1946; signed on 22 July 1946 by the representatives of 61 states (Official Records of the World Health Organization, no. 2, p. 100) and entered into force on 7 April 1948. www.who.int/governance/eb/who_constitution_en.pdf.

14. Moffat, B.M. et al. (2009). A gateway to nature: Teenagers' narratives on smoking marijuana outdoors. *Journal of Environmental Psychology*, 29(1), 86-94.

15. Bottorff, J. et al. (2009, April 23). Relief-oriented use of marijuana by teens. *Substance Abuse Treatment, Prevention, and Policy*, 4(7).

16. Canadian Aids Society. (2006). *Cannabis as therapy for people living with HIV/AIDS : "Our right, our choice."*www.cdnaids.ca/cannabis.

17. COMMON REFERENCE LINKS & LINKS TO MORE INFORMATION INCLUDE:
    1. Cannabiscornercafe.ca : Producer/Publisher
    2. Leafly.com : the world cannabis information resource
    3. Herb.co : An information news resource with a steady growing database of resources and information
    4. CannabisCulture.com
    5. 420pressnews

UPDATED REFERENCES

1. ONLINE STRAIN DATABASES: *With thousands of cannabis strains available, these sites make "getting the details" easy. Search by popularity, time of use, common uses, effects and more. Each offers a unique "presentation" find what you like.*

   - **Leafly:** www.Leafly.ca or www.Leafly.com
   - **CannaConnection:** https://www.cannaconnection.com/strains
   - **WikiLeaf:** www.wikileaf.com/strains

2. Here are a few more cannabis strain databases and a little insight about how they work:

   - HERB Cannabis Strains Database – Strains are categorized by popularity and what is trending at the current time.
     - ➤ http://herb.co
   - SeedFinder – Every strain featured on this site is listed with its seed bank and breeders. The information you can glean from the database include commercial availability, flowering time, height, effects, and aroma.
     - ➤ https://en.seedfinder.eu/
   - 420-101 – Strain names like Platinum Cookies, Blue Dream, and Blueberry Diesel are a few examples of the tempting strains you'll see on 420-101's list. Hover your mouse over a cannabis strain to read its "top 5 medical uses" and reviews.
   - The Cannabis Strain Directory – The website name says it all. An extensive database of highly detailed cannabis strains, this directory's specs, medicinal uses, photos, and the information is sourced from 100+ worldwide seed breeders.
     - ➤ http://thecannabisstraindirectory.com/
   - POTUPEDIA – This medical marijuana strain guide is a comprehensive source and claims to be the largest database of its kind on the web. Each strain featured on the site has a description, explanation, and definition.
     - ➤ http://potupedia.com/
   - Cannaversity – Offering cannabis awareness and education to its readers, Cannaversity has introduced a Cannabis Strain Guide for pot advocates and growers.
     - ➤ https://cannaversity.com/

www.ingramcontent.com/pod-product-compliance
Lightning Source LLC
Chambersburg PA
CBHW031435250726
48656CB00002B/996